Exercises for Doing Mindfully Volume Four

Mindfulness Practices for Persons with Parkinson's Disease

9/3/2014
Parkinsons Recovery
Robert Rodgers PhD

Exercises for Doing Mindfully
Mindfulness Practices for Persons with Parkinson's Disease
Volume Four

Contents

The Parkinsons Recovery Mindfulness Series

Realistically speaking, how can the intense level of stress that aggravates the symptoms of Parkinson's disease be calmed? Better yet, how can they be quieted? My research over the past decade reveals that using your mind to drop the stress level down a notch or two always backfires. When you tell yourself:

- *Settle down!*
- *Take it easy!*
- *Stop being so stressed out!*

The stress level ratchets up, not down. Attempts to force the stress and anxiety levels to adjust downward induce an internally generated stress. They pile more stress on top of an excess of stress that already exists. There are certainly a sufficient number of external generators of stress in every one's life. Why infuse more stress that you create yourself, even with the best of intentions?

If the mind is not a useful technique to reduce stress, what is? The most eloquent answer I have for you is to become more mindful of what is experienced in the present moment. Becoming more mindful shifts you into the experience of the "now" which in itself is less stressful (unless you have been kidnapped by terrorists!).

It is stressful to anticipate events you imagine will occur in the future. The events we imagine rarely happen. Does this ring true for you? We all create unnecessary stress in our lives by how and where we focus our thoughts and attention.

It is stressful to agonize over the past. When we think about the past, we are much more likely to think about unpleasant experiences that induce stress. The past event itself was traumatic enough. Yet, we insist on reliving the trauma over and over again through our memories. It seems some of us just can't get enough stress in our lives.

The problem with upping the ante on stress levels is that – as you well know – symptoms of Parkinson's disease become worse. When you are not as stressed, your symptoms are far less problematic.

I have reached one solid conclusion from my ten years of research on Parkinson's disease. Symptoms will drive you crazy when you are stressed and are far less problematic when stress is under control.

Now, if you can't use your mind to become more mindful (which creates added stress in itself) how in the world can you quiet down a frantic lifestyle? I have concluded that the simplest and most effective solution to reducing stress levels is to become more mindful.

The transformation is possible step by step through these simple exercises you can do anywhere, anytime of the day. The Parkinsons Recovery mindfulness exercises are designed to focus your attention on the present moment as attention on either the past or the future is diverted. A renewed focus on the present moment reduces stress levels. Mindfulness is a lifestyle that will reduce stresses in your life if you set the intention to take a mindfulness practice seriously.

I recommend that you practice each of the exercises for a week or longer. Incorporate each practice into your regular routines and habits. Attempts to do all of the exercises simultaneously will likely induce more stress which – obviously – is contrary to the intent of a successful mindfulness program.

Give each exercise a little time and space. Invite the stresses in your life to dissipate. Allow the experience of each practice to engulf you. In so doing, watch the stresses in your life dip down to new lows along with a concurrent relief of any and all symptoms that you have currently been experiencing.

This volume is one out of nine I have developed to support the recovery of persons who currently experience neurological symptoms. A full listing of the Parkinsons Recovery Mindfulness themes follows:

Exercises for Doing Mindfully
Mindfulness Practices for Persons with Parkinson's Disease
Volume Four

Volume 1: Exercises for Seeing Mindfully

Volume 2: Exercises for Hearing Mindfully

Volume 3: Exercises for Noticing Mindfully

Volume 4: Exercises for Doing Mindfully

Volume 5: Exercises for Eating Mindfully

Volume 6: Exercises for Thinking Mindfully

Volume 7: Exercises for Feeling Mindfully

Volume 8: Exercises for Being Mindfully

Volume 9: Exercises for Intending Mindfully

Robert Rodgers, PhD

Parkinsons Recovery

www.parkinsonsrecovery.me

Olympia, Washington

Mindful Driving

The Mindfulness Challenge of this week focuses attention on driving. If you currently do not drive a car or a vehicle but rather ride in cars, all of my suggestions will still apply to you although you are not actually driving yourself.

I have a confession to make at the outset. I have been practicing this particular exercise for several months now. It has been a true challenge for me to convert my normal practice of scatterbrain driving to one of mindful driving. What I discovered for myself (before I decided to issue this challenge to you) is that I consider driving to be a secondary function. I don't wish to "waste" any of my precious time, so while I am driving I am planning out my next activity of the day. I was surprised and shocked to discover that there would be blocks of time, sometimes five minutes - sometimes ten, when I was literally somewhere else. I was not attentive to where I was at the moment or for that matter where I was headed.

I converted this habit of mindless driving to a habit of mindful driving, but only after I realized that I typically consider driving to be a secondary and unimportant function. The task is anything but that, especially if you want to avert accidents and other serious problems. When I say mindful driving what exactly does that entail?

6

Pay close attention to every aspect of the experience of getting into the vehicle and sitting down wherever you elect to sit. Become totally and completely aware of how your body is positioned in the seat including where your legs are positioned. Does your body feel as though that is the right placement for you in terms of the height of the seat are sitting in?

> *How does it feel when you take the key and insert it into the ignition, if in fact that's the way your car works? Does the metal feel cold or slimy or wet?*

> *How does it feel when you put your hands on your steering wheel? Is it sticky perhaps? Is it warm or is it too cold?*

As you turn the car on, be mindful. Pay attention to how the engine is running. Treat it as a child.

> *How you feeling today, dear?*

Your engine will tell you what is really up in the moment. As you begin to engage that journey of the drive look, notice and be totally attentive to every nuance of the driving experience.

Be aware of persons that may be riding bikes or walking on the side of the road. What do you do when you see such obstructions? Do you consider them to be just that? What do you do when a driver nudges up behind you wanting to travel 20 more miles an hour than you are driving? As you look in our rear-view mirror you happen to notice that they are two-inches from your bumper. What do you do when that happens? What is your reaction?

Become mindful of each moment as you drive. Become aware of all the motions, all reactions and all thoughts that are connected to the driving experience in the moment.

- *Do you typically drive right at the speed limit, below the speed limit or faster than the speed limit?*
- *What are the thoughts that drive your decision?*
- *Are you someone who has the thought that the police never stop a person who drives less than ten miles over the speed limit and so you choose to always drive ten miles faster?*

Become aware then of whatever thoughts and feelings you experience as you drive moment to moment.

The most important aspect of this challenge is of course to be present to the moment, unlike myself who tended to space out and be totally unaware of what I was doing. It is true that as the years pass by, driving can become very automatic. It is also true that we avert potentially dangerous and life-threatening accidents for ourselves and others when we are observant of traffic behind, in front and to each side of the vehicle.

Being mindful of the driving experience also enriches that experience. We have an opportunity to observe all of the beauty that we actually pass by such as the flowers and the trees. We actually get to observe and experience the smells, the feeling of what it is like to ride in that car and be vibrated as we bounce here and there. It is also exhilarating to be attentive to the different road surfaces and how the driving experience shifts when that road surface becomes smooth or bumpy in transition.

Notice your habit of driving. Mindfulness means being present in the moment. When you drive you are not being mindful when you are planning your evening. You are not being mindful when you are evaluating something you might have said to a person earlier in the day. Live in the present moment. When you live in the present your life is enriched immeasurably. Most importantly stress dissolves like an ice-cream cone in the sunshine.

Deeper Implications Behind Mindful Driving

What are the deeper implications for becoming mindful and attentive of driving a vehicle or riding in a vehicle? Driving a car or riding in one has a direct analogy to the journey of recovering from Parkinson's disease. Permit me to explain.

When driving, it is almost always the case that we have a very clear and precise destination in mind. Of course that is not always the case, but almost always if we are in the car either driving or riding we are going somewhere. On your journey of recovery from the symptoms of Parkinson's disease, my question to you is:

Where are you headed on your journey?

Is the end goal to see a release of the tension in your right thigh or an elimination of a tremor in your left arm? Do you set for yourself a goal that is actually one that has a negative connotation? In other words, do you desire as an end goal a symptom that is currently annoying to suddenly disappear and dissolve?

Consider your possible experience with driving to two very different destinations. The first destination is a concert by a musical group that you truly love. You are going to be very motivated to get there. You are going to be energetic. You are going to be happy. You are going to be

10

exhilarated because once you arrive, you will enter the concert hall and experience something that you truly and genuinely treasure.

Contrast that destination with a destination of driving to a billing center which has wrongly charged you $125 dollars on your internet bill. What is it like to experience driving to that destination? We all are different of course but if you are like me, I'm thinking to myself,

> *"Do I really have to spend my time and energy going to this office and appear in person to straighten this out? I'm really upset and angry about this. I don't want to waste my day spending my time driving over there and solving something that shouldn't have happened in the first place, blah, blah, blah, blah, blah, blah."*

Does that sound familiar? Do you get a feeling for the contrast between those two destinations? It is really very similar to a destination and a goal that you might set for yourself when it comes to recovery. If the intention (and end state goal) is to eliminate a symptom, that is fine and good but it is certainly not anything that you will ever look forward to.

Why not set an end state goal that does serve and fulfill your true passion? Only you know what that might be of course. Part of our journey through life is to act on our passions.

Speaking personally, I have realized recently that one of my passions is writing short stories. I stopped and thought to myself,

> "I need to start writing short stories because I love it!"

It has taken me quite a few years to actually make that statement and engage that behavior. What is your fondest passion that you have put on the shelf for reasons that more than likely do not make a lot of sense? Let me just give one example of a possible passion that perhaps one or even more of you might have.

Suppose your passion is to paint. You want to begin to paint again. You have some challenges, some difficulties with painting now given that some of the symptoms are making painting more challenging. The end goal is to paint. Once the goal is established, a goal that does have energetic juice, consider the journey to be a lot like driving where you are attentive and present to each and every moment.

The end goal is to paint but you no longer have any paint brushes. You make a decision to acquire some paint brushes. So, you get in your car and mindfully drive to the art store. Perhaps this is all you can accomplish for this day or this week or even this month. It is a small segment of a very long journey, but you have a clear idea of the end goal. The end goal is to return to what you truly love, which is painting.

Consider what end state goals you set for yourself. Once they are set ask yourself,

> *"Am I rushing like a mad person to achieve that goal just as I drive like a mad person to get to the destinations that I set for myself?"*

Chances are there is little difference between the two.

When you recognize and acknowledge your habits of driving, you will also have at your fingertips important information about your own approach to recovering from whatever symptoms you might currently experience. Becoming mindful of this journey to achieve your end goal (to manifest your passions) means you are attentive and mindful to each and every moment of the journey. Yes, the journey might last a month or two months or even three or four months before you are even in a position to begin to start painting. Each and every day, each and every hour, each and every second you were attentive and mindful to what you needed to do for yourself to be in a position where yes, you could finally manifest your passion and – in my example, paint.

In summary, ask:

What are my end goal states?

What are my passions?

What am I driving to achieve?

Do I simply want to eliminate pain and discomfort, or do I desire something more?

How am I getting to my destination in the most important vehicle of all - my body? Am I rushing, or am I driving on my journey mindfully?

Make It Better

My Mindfulness Challenge this week involves taking a number of small, tiny steps or actions accompanied with a reflection of your reactions, thoughts and feelings to taking those actions. What actions am I going to suggest that you take? It is really quite simple.

In every place that you find yourself, look around and see what tiny small action you can take to make that place a little bit better. What do I mean exactly?

- *Perhaps you are in the kitchen. You notice that there is a bit of mess on the counter top. This may be your habit, but if not – simply wipe that little mess on the counter top up. It takes about 10 or 15 seconds at most; typically something that you may not do by manner of routine.*
- *Perhaps you notice that in the bedroom there is a piece of paper on the carpet. Pick up the paper. Dispose of it either in the trash or put it where it actually belongs.*
- *Perhaps you are walking on the sidewalk outside while taking your afternoon walk. You notice that there is a paper bag on the side of the road. Pick up the paper bag. When you find a place to dispose of it, dispose of it.*

I could of course give endless examples but the idea is to leave each place that you find yourself just a tiny bit better than it was when you first arrived.

"Make it Better" is the idea here. Anything goes. Anything that you can do to improve a situation counts. Enjoy this challenge but be sure to acknowledge every feeling and thought that you have when you do just what I am suggesting, whatever those thoughts and feelings might be. There will probably be a long list of reactions that you may have. These thoughts and reactions are rich information for you to work with as this particular challenge unfolds.

Implications Behind Making It Better

How is the challenge been going to make each situation you find yourself a little bit better?

- *Have you done it?*
- *Have you enjoyed it?*
- *Have you hated it?*
- *Have you struggled with this particular challenge?*

Some of you may have been anticipating that this is actually a bit of a prissy challenge. By prissy I mean that perhaps you were thinking I was going to say something to the effect of,

> *"Well, if each person just did exactly what you have been doing these last few days, make each situation just a little bit better, wouldn't the world at large be a whole lot more wonderful and beautiful place to live?"*

All of this is true certainly, but this rationale is not the underlying motivation for my suggesting that you make each and every situation just a little bit better.

There are actually two important and compelling reasons to invite you to continue with this challenge for the rest of the week. The first reason is really quite simple. You look around at a situation and often times we see incredible problems. There is:

- *Trash*
- *Mess*
- *Disarray*
- *Chaos*

We think to ourselves,

> *"Oh my heavens, this particular situation is absolutely chaotic. It is horrible. Who in the world could ever set this straight? There is no way that I could do anything about all the trash people throw out of the cars. The problem is overwhelming. "*

I often have that thought when I drive down the highway and see the trash that has been thrown on the roadway.

Isn't that, I ask you, the very same type of thinking that rattles around your mind at times when you reflect on symptoms you might be experiencing? Might I suggest to you there is really little difference between thoughts about trash on the roadways and thoughts about symptoms?

When lots of symptoms begin to flare it is normal to begin to think,

"This is overwhelming. There is absolutely no way any of this can be reversed. I am discouraged. I am depressed. It does not even matter what action I take. It will not make a hill of beans difference anyway!"

Does that set of thoughts sound familiar to you? The reality is really just the reverse. Symptoms begin to reverse when we take tiny, small steps - when we take actions that may seem to be of little consequence. If we simply get stuck and become couch potatoes, symptoms will become even more overwhelming.

Individuals who find they succeed in reversing their symptoms take tiny, little actions each and every day. It might only take a minute or two or five minutes, but when you begin to take "baby steps on your journey down the road to recovery, it will make a huge a difference in how you actually feel throughout the rest of the day if not the rest of the week.

Tiny steps create small wins. Yes, it is insurmountable to think of what you need to do today to reverse any and all symptoms you might be experiencing. I agree that as an end goal, this challenge is overwhelming.

That's not the point! The point is to feel a little bit better today. You do that by taking a small action.

There is a second underlying reason for this particular challenge that may come as a bit of a surprise to you. You have been monitoring your reactions and thoughts when you have been cleaning up for others because of course this exercise entails cleaning up the mess, not only your own mess but the messes of other individuals–family members, loved ones, perhaps even strangers. I can tell you what some of my reactions have been to this exercise.

I walk into the kitchen, I see a horrible mess. The kids have been there last night. Okay, okay what's my choice? Do I tell them,

> "Get in here and clean it up!"?

Or do I say,

> "Forget it. I'm just going to do it myself"?

What do I feel? Resentment. Then as I begin to clean up the dishes I begin to think to myself,

> "When is this going to be over? When are these kids going to grow up? My goodness, I don't know how much longer I can live with this!"

Feelings of anger and resentment begin to surge inside my body. Your reactions may be very different but you get the point.

Of course there is a huge range of reactions that all of us will have depending on what the circumstance actually is - especially when we're dealing with strangers. We see something that has been thrown on the side of the road and all of a sudden surging up inside our physical body can be the feeling of rage. Why in the world are people out there willing to do such horrible things like eat a sandwich and put the residue on the side of the road? Yuk.

As we monitor all of those feelings, I suggest that these too are all of the same thoughts and feelings that are accompanied with anyone who currently experiences neurological symptoms associated with the diagnosis of Parkinson's disease. Aren't I right? Isn't there resentment?

> "Why in the world did I have to get this? My God, I don't know of anybody else that has it?"

Isn't there anger towards your body?

> "You're not working! Give me a break would you get on board please?"

I suggest that all of those feelings that emerge when you do this harmless little task of making every situation a little bit better are similar to the emotions and feelings that are associated with how you feel about symptoms that you currently experience. Are those feelings and thoughts in your best and highest good? Answer is no.

- *They are not helping you.*
- *They are not helping your body.*
- *They are not helping your mind.*
- *They are not helping your soul.*
- *They are dragging you down deep into the gutter.*

The idea of course is to recognize those feelings and thoughts when they emerge. We all have them. We can't stop them. But then say,

> *"Oh right, of course I'm resentful! Why don't I just put that resentment to rest for now? I really do not need to expend any energy on that feeling right now."*

One of the strategies that I use often when I identify a feeling that I know is not in my best and highest good is to say,

> *"Okay, I'm human, I have a right to feel that resentment, what I'm going to do is put it up in the cupboard and I'll shut the door of the cupboard. I can take the resentment out of the cupboard tomorrow or next week if I really want to and feel as though I need to."*

The magic of my strategy of course is that I never remember to open up the cupboard and take out the feeling of resentment for additional examination. OK. I realize this is a pretty silly approach but it works for me! I stop having the resentment seethe throughout all the cells in my body. This makes room for feelings and thoughts that do serve my best and highest good.

Continue with this particular challenge for the rest of the week. You may (by way of habit) do this anyway, or you may decide to continue doing it after the week expires. Notice this week each and every feeling and thought that emerges when you take each action to "Make it Better".

1.   *Recognize it is a familiar thought or feeling.*

2.   *Recognize it is tied to sustaining symptoms. .*

3.   *Put it in the cupboard.*

4.   *Shut the door.*

5.   *Activate feelings and thoughts that will promote a reversal of whatever symptoms.*

Begin taking those steps that are necessary to help your body heal. The body is a miracle. It knows exactly what needs to happen in order to come back into full balance and harmony.

Breathe and Drink Water

There is no doubt about it. When neurological symptoms flare we all furiously begin to search for options that offer the promise of quick relief. We furiously engage our minds to understand what is causing the symptoms. We eagerly search for options that provide temporary relief or even reverse the symptoms.

In other words, we are continuously in our minds

- **Thinking**
- **Thinking**
- **Thinking**

We are thinking each and every moment of our waking lives. True healing lies in a place that resides deep inside the cells of our body - not in our minds. How do we access this unique gateway to healing? Two options are sure bets.

The first is to hydrate your body; to hydrate your cells. Many people do not drink enough water. The second is to breath, to give those cells enough oxygen.

These two therapies are both simple. They are free. They are easy to do. You can activate each of these therapies at any point in time during the day. No doctor is required to write a prescription. These two approaches will

24

potentially yield enormous returns if practiced on a regular basis.

My invitation for you this week is quite simple. Several times during the day, especially when you are having negative and hurtful thoughts that are rattling through your mind over and over, stop. Take three breaths - as deep as is comfortable.

When you breathe allow yourself, just for a moment, to become aware of colors, sounds, touches and smells, all of which we are often ignorant of when we are in our heads. Take three long and delicious breaths at least three times during the day.

1. **Stop. Take a slow breath in and out.**
2. **Take a second breath in and out.**
3. **Take a third breath in and out.**

Then, take a sip of water. I am talking here a simple task that will consume no more than 20 or 30 seconds, three times a day.

Notice how everything shifts. Notice how your awareness deepens. Notice how you reach that place deep inside your cells, the place of true and genuine and profound healing. This is the place where neurological symptoms are reversed. No money is required. No prescription is needed. Simply practice breathing and sipping water three times—three times a day.

Deeper Meaning Behind Oxygen and Water

You might well be wondering why it so useful and productive and helpful to stop three times a day and take three breaths. We are always thinking, not only when are awake, but when we are asleep. We are pondering past pains and past traumas, trying to make sense out of how in the world those traumas could have occurred. We are planning future events; the next ten minutes, the next day, the next week, the coming year. We are, as it turns out, focusing our attention either on the past or on the future and not where life is really at—the present.

We never, as it turns out, really give our thinking minds a break. You are probably thinking,

> *"But I sleep and my mind rests then."*

I am afraid not my friends. When we sleep we dream. Our minds are actually more active when we are asleep than we are awake. We may not remember the thinking that occurred when we were asleep, but I assure you our minds are overly-active when we sleep.

The question then becomes:

> **When do we really ever give our thinking minds a break, a rest?**

26

Some people who practice doing daily meditations do give their minds a rest but a successful mediation practices demands practice and discipline. Such persons are in the minority. A practice of meditation using breath as the focus is difficult. What is this difficulty? The mind gets scared and frightened, afraid that we intend to undo its purpose.

The mind convinces most people they are not doing their meditation practice correctly or that they are being cajoled into doing something they really did not want to do in the first place. They stop meditating. Has this been your experience too?

The underlying meaning of taking three breaths here and there throughout the day is to trick your mind (and your subconscious) into becoming acclimated to the pleasure of taking a short rest from thinking now and then.

The mind actually does like to rest, so we simply invite it to do so over the course of 20 or 30 seconds throughout the day. Taking three breaths three times a day is an easy way to break into a mindfulness meditation practice if that happens to be the direction you are interested in pursuing.

Three breaths also give you oxygen. If you really monitor how much you breathe, you will be quite amazed to discover that there are times when there is very little if any oxygen coming into your body. If your cells don't get oxygen, you certainly aren't going to have very much energy. Taking three breaths at least three times throughout each day will actually enhance your energy level. Think about adding a glass of water to that particular activity and you'll bolster your energy level five-fold.

Three breaths, three times a day.

- It is free to do.
- It is easy to do.
- It is relaxing.
- It is enjoyable.

And why not add a sip of water for an extra energy boost. Water does not have the side effects of energy drinks!

This simple action shifts your attention to that deeper place of profound and genuine healing—the place where it is possible to reverse neurological symptoms that are being aggravated by an over-active neurological system. When all of your energy resides in your head - from your thinking self - it is very challenging indeed to access all of the other senses.

Three breaths take you to a place where you are able to activate an awareness of your immediate surroundings as you notice the:

- **Colors,**
- **Sounds,**
- **Sights,**
- **Smells,**
- **Sensations.**

It takes you away from a place in our minds where we tend to live all of our lives. Enrich your life; give your body an opportunity to reverse those neurological symptoms by taking three simple breaths several times a day.

Healing Touch

Whether we currently experience the neurological symptoms associated with Parkinson's disease or not, we all have aches, pains and disturbances throughout our body from day to day:

- *A toe that aches today*
- *A knee that is troublesome tomorrow*
- *A shoulder that become tight tonight*
- *An arm that emits pain over the weekend*
- *A finger that happens to be painful next week*

There are many reactions that we have when our body sends out signals of discomfort. One of those reactions is to make a visit to the doctor who will prescribe medications or perhaps even surgery. That is one solution and it works well for some people.

A second solution is to get furious at that part of your body that is sending out signals of angst. We can always fuss away at our body. We can always be angry at it when it is not doing for us what we want it to do in the moment.

There is a third response that I invite you to mindfully attend to this week. When you notice that your body is sending out some signal of discomfort, for example, a left knee that happens to ache or a right shoulder that happens to be somewhat painful, instead of going to the doctor – though that might be important and necessary – and instead of beating-up on your body, try a third strategy. Take one of your hands and place that hand on the place that is calling out to you for attention.

For example, if it is your left knee that happens to be troubling you today, place your left hand on that left knee. That is all you have to do, nothing else. Just place your hand on your left knee. If it is your right shoulder that is bothering you in the moment, place your left hand on your right shoulder. Just hold your hand there.

Finally, and perhaps mostly helpful is when you are going to sleep at night, do a scan of your body. Ask what body parts happen to be calling out to you in the moment with some degree of distress. Take the same simple action.

Place a hand over on that shoulder, stomach, hip, thigh or knee. If it happens to be your foot you can obviously put yourself in a position where you can place your hand over your foot. Make it so that you are totally comfortable, so much so that you can go to sleep with your hand on that body part that is troubling you.

I emphasize, nothing else is required—no thoughts are needed of any type. Simply place your hand on the body part that is calling out for attention. It is called "healing touch." No workshops are required. No special skills are necessary. It is not necessary to read any instructional books – just touch the place on your body that is calling out for a little loving attention. Leave your hand in the same position as long as possible.

Apply "healing touch" whenever the occasion calls for it this week during the day, but especially as you are going to sleep at night.

Try it. You will like it.

Long Term Implications for Healing Touch

From 1999 until 2003, I attended a healing school. The school presented many challenging lessons that needed to be learned; many of them involved personal processing, but many were also healing techniques. We would learn a healing technique each time we went to school in either New York or Florida. The new healing technique required considerable focus, discipline and of course we had to be evaluated on the extent to which we learned it. It was a rigorous training program.

The most useful healing technique that I learned over the four years of training is "healing touch" as I have described it.

- No special training in healing techniques is necessary.
- No trips to New York or Florida are necessary.
- No discipline, focus or intention is necessary.

Results can be quite marvelous indeed. You can literally take your hand and place it anywhere on your body that is troubling. Relief will be forthcoming.

Instead of beating up on our body, instead of being angry it is not working the way it is supposed to work according to our expectations and standards – we pay attention to it.

We listen to our body and place a hand on the body part that is calling out for attention.

By placing your hand on the particular place on your body that needs attention, you call in the frequencies that are needed for healing the discomfort. Don't ask me to explain how or why this works. I really don't have a clue. All I know is it works. I know it works because I've used this every night since I've learned the technique.

- *It is easy to do.*
- *It is fun.*
- *It will console that place on your body that is calling out to you for attention.*
- *It is soothing.*
- *It helps bring your body back in to balance.*

Most obviously, instead of having thought forms that have very low frequency and that are disastrously judgmental – instead, you have a tender, loving response to your body that in reality is working beautifully.

If you are like me, now that you know about this healing technique, if you have any place on your body that calls out for attention - you will be placing that hand there now and forever more.

Leave No Trace

The physical setting where we reside, eat, live and enjoy our life is symbolic of our inner health. Look around where you are currently sitting or standing right now. Are the physical surroundings tidy, are they orderly? You might say,

> *"I've never been a tidy or orderly person. It doesn't make any sense to me to lead a life that is totally tidy and wrapped up. I'm just not that type of person."*

When we clean up the clutter that surrounds our life, we allow the life force to move through our bodies. We gain energy.

If there is significant clutter that surrounds us where we eat, live and work, it is likely that our life force will be stifled and stymied. There are two ways to approach this challenge. The first approach is to say

> *"Once I begin feeling better, once my health returns, once I have reversed the symptoms that I have been experiencing, then I'll be able to clean up the mess in my living room, office, kitchen, in my bedroom. I'll get to work on that when I feel better."*

A second approach is to reverse the thinking process. You acknowledge,

- **"No, I don't have a lot of energy today."**
- **"No, I'm not feeling particularly well."**
- **"Yes, my symptoms are in my face."**
- **"But, I'm going to simply begin cleaning up the clutter in my life."**

Guess what will happen? You'll get more energy. Your life force will begin to flow through every cell of your body. Your energy will begin to sizzle.

The mindfulness challenge this week is to leave no trace in a place of choosing in your home. This particular place could be a kitchen, a bedroom, an office or even a corner of an office. For example, we continuously eat and oftentimes leave the dishes in the sink without washing them. If your choice is to focus your challenge of the week on the kitchen do the following.

When you use dishes, wash them immediately. Do not leave the dishes in the sink. Do not expect someone else will clean them up. Do not say to yourself

"I'll attend to that tomorrow."

The challenge of the week is to be mindful of everything that you use. Honor it. Respect its sacredness. Celebrate the value that it gives to you whether that object is a fork, a spoon, a knife, a plate, a toothbrush, a pencil, a pen or papers.

To summarize, the challenge of the week is to focus on keeping a corner in your home or office tidy throughout the week. Leave no trace in the space of your choosing. When you make a mess, clean it up immediately so that when you leave that space, you leave no trace. It is as if you were never there. Nobody would know you were there, not even a professional detective.

Deeper Implications Behind Leaving No Trace

What has been your experience with tidying up a corner of your house or office? Reflect on your experience. Have you been thinking as you've tidied up,

> *"This is sure taking a lot of time. I'd much rather be doing A or B or C."*

Perhaps you were thinking,

> *"Is this really something that is going to help? I could really defer this particular activity until tomorrow."*

As you have been tidying up have you thought -

> *"Oh, I really need to go and do that other, important task that I promised myself I would do right now."*

In other words, as you were attending to the challenge of tidying up, were you actually living in the future or the past and not the present? Were you actually not attentive to the experience of what it means to put everything back in its proper place?

The challenge of the week is to invite you to reflect on your reactions doing something that you typically would not do. There is, however, a deeper and much more profound implication to this particular assignment.

Our egos are extremely effective at sabotaging our intent to get well. We have all sorts of rationales that we use for why we should not attend to doing what it is that we well know will help us feel significantly better.

How many times have you said,

> *"Yes, yes I know I need to exercise today. I know I'll feel better but I just don't feel up to it."*

How many times have you said that to yourself? My hand is raised. I use that rationale all the time. Or how about,

> *"Oh, I really should go out for a walk but it's drizzling outside. I don't want to walk in the rain. It might make me sick."*

You see, we have very intricate and extensive rationales that we use for why it is that we cannot attend to the tasks and the duties that we know will help us feel better.

How about eating healthy food? How many times have you said,

> *"Well, I don't feel like eating that fresh, live food today. I think I'd much rather have steak, potatoes and macaroni and cheese."*

Yes, that is yummy food for the stomach. For some people it is comfort food. But is it really going to help you feel better? You know the answer.

> *"No, I'm not going to feel better if I eat unhealthy food."*

The challenge then is to acknowledge the times when we concoct seemingly rational reasons why we should not be doing what is in our best and highest good.

- We really do know what we need to do to feel better.
- We really do know what we need to do to help ourselves reverse symptoms.

Yet, we persist with the same bad habits that undo our ability to recover and become symptom-free.

Becoming mindful of physical tasks like leaving no trace is a golden opportunity to transfer those same rationales over to our decision-making about what we must do for ourselves to heal. One common rationale is to say

> *"I have to work. I have to make money. I really don't have time to be able to go to these appointments with these health care providers."*

Does that rationale sound familiar to you? You see, it is the same as deciding you need to leave the dishes in the sink.

Enjoy continuing your assignment and accepting the challenge to become totally and completely mindful of tidying up. When you tidy up that sink, when you tidy up that bathroom or whatever corner of the house you've chosen to focus on, you actually transfer the same skill set over to being able to take the actions that are needed to tidy up all of the imbalances that are currently present in your body.

It's an approach that is positive.

- **It will guarantee that a strong life force will begin to flow through every cell of your body.**
- **It will ensure that you are focused on the moment.**
- **It will guarantee that you will act on the intuitions that you have about what is necessary to begin feeling better.**

Have fun as you continue tidying up that corner of the house that has been full of clutter for all too long.

Use Your Non-Dominant Hand

I have a warning before I now explain the mindfulness challenge for the week. This week's challenge will take an additional 15 to 30 minutes of your time every day. It is, in a way then, indirectly a lesson in learning to be more patient. Here is the challenge if indeed you wish to accept it.

The challenge is, first of all, to acknowledge which of your two hands is the non-dominant hand. One of the hands for most people is the hand you use most frequently. The other hand is the hand you use less frequently. Which of your two hands is the non-dominant hand? The challenge is to put that non-dominant hand to greater use in three very specific tasks I will now describe.

Task One: Brushing your teeth. Instead of using the hand that you usually use, use your non-dominant hand when you brush your teeth.

Task Two: Combing your hair. Instead of using your dominant hand as you customarily would do while combing and brushing your hair, use your non-dominant hand to comb your hair this week.

Task Three: Eat with you non-dominant hand. This is one task that may require extra time and concentration. Place your eating utensil in your non-dominant hand as your eat one entire meal each day during the week.

I fully realize that you will be particularly challenged this week if your non-dominant hand happens to be a hand where there is tremoring in which case it will be particularly difficult and frustrating to use your non-dominant hand for any of the three tasks. I offer one suggestion for being able to activate energy in a hand that may also be associated with some motor dysfunction.

With your intention, take the strong and vibrant energy from the other side of your body where the symptoms are not as prevalent or troublesome and - using your intention - shift the strong and vibrant energy over to your non-dominant hand. You can accomplish the transfer quickly and swiftly just as a martial artist would shift energy in their body from one side to the next. Here is the sequence:

1. Take a deep breath in
2. Place the back of your tongue up against the top of your throat
3. Exhale your breath out quickly you (with your intention) shift the energy to your non-dominant hand.

This particular exhale sounds something like "Haah...phuh!" That's what it sounds like. It is a very quick burst.

When you are eating with family members, you might want to explain this is just a fun way that you are experimenting with to shift energy from one side of your body to the other. It sounds rather ridiculous I'm sure to many of you, but it actually does work. You can shift the energy and balance out the right and the left sides of your body using this simple technique that is a standard technique used in martial arts practice.

Continue to practice using your non-dominant hand whether it might be a hand on the side of your body that is creating motor difficulties or not. It really does not matter. What you want to do is to exercise the golden and precious practice of mindfulness. Bring your thoughts to the present moment. Live in the now, not a second before and not a second after. Using your non-dominant hand requires your full attention so that you can get the tasks that need to be done of brushing your teeth, combing your hair and eating at least one meal a day.

May you have delicious fun with this activity all week long as you practice the art of mindfulness using a hand that is under-utilized. In so doing may the stress in your life vanish forever more.

Deeper Meaning Behind Using Your Non-Dominant Hand

What in the world is the meaning behind doing a silly task like using your non-dominant hand? I interview hundreds and hundreds of individuals every year that have the symptoms of Parkinson's and ask the question,

> *"What is it that helps you the most to get sustained relief from your symptoms?"*

An answer I frequently hear reported back to me is the following.

> *"I've discovered that really helps is to simply slow down. Instead of trying to move as quickly as I moved when I was ten years old, I've learned to take my movements mindfully. When I do this I've discovered that my movements become smoother and much more graceful."*

Mindfulness really is the ticket to sustaining true balance and harmony. You have to slow everything down to be mindful.

How is the exercise of using your non-dominant hand coming along? Have you been so frustrated because it has taken so much time to brush your teeth or comb your hair or eat a meal with a non-dominant hand that you've just skipped a few days? Perhaps you decided that you just do

45

not have enough time in the day to fuss around with doing such a silly task like using a hand that is not your best one?

You see this task helps you realize the true degree to which you tend to be impatient. Acknowledge whatever degree of impatience you might have experienced. Honor the value that is inherent in bringing your consciousness to the present moment.

When you experience life as it unfolds in the moment, the entire experience of impatience becomes irrelevant. The experience of the moment is all that counts. Each and every moment becomes magical. Living in the moment has welcome consequences. Imbalances that are currently present in the body can potentially be resolved because stress is not on the center stage.

One golden lesson from this exercise is that it affords you the opportunity to be more compassionate. Why? As you become frustrated with being unable to do tasks that are much easier when you use your dominant hand, you transcend back into the time long ago when you were a child, when those particular tasks were much more challenging. This particular task then, you see, teaches the golden lesson to have more compassion for yourself.

How many times have you been frustrated with the fact you:

1. can't move or
2. can't talk or
3. can't function or
4. can't think or
5. can't swallow?

Everyone has symptoms of one type or another but if you currently have a diagnosis of Parkinson's, some symptoms are truly frustrating. When a symptom rears its ugly head, what is your gut reaction?

- To get frustrated with yourself?
- To get upset?
- To go into fear about the long term consequences?

Hum, that is interesting because you are not having very much compassion for yourself.

I have a statement to make that I think is pretty universally true of many individuals with Parkinson's. You're really good at helping other people and being compassionate for the struggles of others. But, you rarely extend that same compassion to yourself. My guess is that you are awfully hard on yourself.

Switch that around. Even out the compassion you have to offer to others. Be just as compassionate to yourself and to your own struggles as you are to the struggles of others.

Do a little calculation of the total compassion you offer to others. Add the compassion you offer to family members to the compassion you offer to strangers to the compassion you offer to friends. What is the total compassion index that you offer to others every day? It probably has enough energetic charge to light up an entire city.

Now, take that total energetic surge of compassion you extend so generously to others and turn it inward. Be open to becoming more compassionate to yourself.

Delight in the magic of each and every moment without agonizing over what has happened to you or your family in the past. The past is over. There is nothing you can do to change it. Fears about the future are almost always unfounded. All such worries are entirely irrelevant to what is happening now in the present. Bring yourself to the magic of the moment as you continue undertaking the challenge of using your non-dominant hand for the rest of the week.

Another revelation that you will discover is, yes, it is very difficult to do these exercises: brushing your teeth, combing your hair and eating with a non-dominant hand in the beginning. But guess what? It gets easier. You get

48

better at it if you will continue doing these simple exercises not just for the rest of the week, but next week and the weeks to follow.

You see, it is possible to be able to get sustained relief from the symptoms of Parkinson's by giving yourself a heavy dose of compassion, by being patient to what is happening in the moment and by being totally and completely present to yourself and others.

- *May you have fun*
- *May you enjoy this exercise*
- *May you invite others to join in the fun for it can be truly revealing .*

It will transform your attitudes toward yourself and toward the possibility of recovering fully and completely.

Anonymous Acts of Kindness

My invitation for you this week is to be totally sneaky and secretive. Doesn't just hearing that give you a burst of energy? We were certainly secretive and sneaky when we were kids. When we become adults most people tend to be honest and open and want to be forthright.

This week, however, adopt a more secretive life. My invitation and challenge is to commit an anonymous act of kindness each day. Let me emphasize the word anonymous. My guess is that many of you commit many, many acts of kindness every day to others and hopefully to yourself.

The difference is that these acts of kindness need to be anonymous. No one should know that you actually committed any particular act of kindness on their behalf.

I must warn you at the outset. This is not as easy as it sounds. This requires a bit of planning the night before. Please put a little notebook beside your bed. Before you retire for the night plan out exactly what act of kindness you will commit the next day. Feel free to sneaky and cleaver in your plans.

Keep in mind that you do not want to be caught. You don't want anyone to realize,

50

"Ah, I figured it out. You were the one who did it. Well, thanks a lot."

That is not the idea here. The idea is that all acts of kindness that you commit must be anonymous and secret. That is why it takes a little advance planning to succeed with this mindfulness exercise.

I'm going to give you now some examples of what anonymous acts of kindness might look like. Obviously the list is endless. I could presents thousands of examples, but in the end you will have to come up with your own ideas of what would give you a burst of energy in committing an anonymous act of kindness that has meaning for you.

For example, you could:

- *Wash dishes that are dirty for someone else. Of course if you live in a household where it is obvious you were the one who did it, that particular act is not going to be anonymous.*
- *Pick up some trash during a walk in your neighborhood. Nobody is going to know that you actually did that.*
- *Make an anonymous donation to a charity that you treasure and relish.*
- *Leave a health food candy bar on a co-worker's desk when no one else is looking.*
- *Send an anonymous note of appreciation and thanks to someone who was particularly helpful,*

51

though you obviously don't want to be clear about what they did specifically.

- *Answer a question (that you happen to have the answer to) on the internet, but do that anonymously.*
- *Send flowers to a friend – what a thrill it is to receive flowers and you have no idea who sent them!*
- *Plant a tree in your yard for a loved one who may be particularly challenged or troubled this week.*
- *Send a prayer in your thoughts as you pass by a stranger. Your prayer could be: "May you find endless joy and happiness today."*

Please remember the rules of this kindness mindfulness invitation this week.

1. **It needs to be an act of kindness; that is probably not going to be hard to fulfill.**
2. **The act of kindness needs to be anonymous. Nobody can figure out that you actually committed the deed.**

The end result promises to:

- *Open up those blocked energy channels and meridians throughout your body.*
- *Strengthen your energy field.*
- *Actualize your divine essence.*
- *Come into your full power.*

52

One of the ways to accomplish these ambitious goals is to be mindful in committing anonymous acts of kindness. May you have a magnificent week as you dole out random acts of kindness that are entirely anonymous.

Deeper Meaning Behind Anonymous Acts of Kindness

The purpose of each week's mindfulness exercise is to take us out of our head and to take us out of our ego into the mysterious glory and wonder of being in the present moment as we live life to the fullest. You have heard this many times. We cannot undo the past and we cannot know the future. The best we can do is to be fully present in the moment.

What is the deeper meaning that underlies the assignment this week to commit random acts of kindness that are anonymous? Why not let people know exactly what you did? Isn't that more honest you might ask? Well here's the reason.

When we actually do something for someone else, there is a lot of mental gobbledygook that underpins that decision. I do it myself all the time. For example, I decide to do something for a friend because they have done something for me recently. I think to myself,

> *"You know, I need to balance this out. They keep inviting us to dinner, we need to exchange that invitation and invite them to dinner. They know that they invited us to dinner and of course we know that we need to invite them."*

54

Don't get me wrong. There is nothing wrong with this thinking. It is obviously important to have an even exchange of giving and taking with friends. But this thinking also shifts us away from being totally and completely in the moment - of relishing the wonder and the glory of being able to do something for another person. Our thoughts can always give us a logical rationale for why we are doing what we do for others.

Acts of kindness then may actually be on their face, an act of kindness, but underneath there may be an expectation of some giveback, some return. For example,

> *"I'll do this for you and now, because you owe something to me, you're going to have to do something for me, which is what I've been asking for all along."*

Again, let me emphasize, there's nothing wrong with this rationale, but it does take us out of being totally and completely present in the moment.

You will experience a surge of energy when you commit anonymous acts of kindness. They have a purity about them that offers a rush of joy and exhilaration. There are no expectations of a pay back. There is no thought that this is something you are doing to even out the score with another person. The act on its face is simply a pure and unadulterated act of kindness that comes from your heart.

This invitation - if you have chosen to accept it - is quite exhilarating in itself because it requires that you invent ways to be totally and completely in the present moment. You do that and you do not have any entanglement with your ego or your mind. You do not think about the past. You do not anticipate or worry about the future. When you commit your act of kindness you are totally and completely in the present.

Some acts of kindness require that you be more attentive to the present or else you are going to get caught. You have to be very grounded and centered when you commit these acts or else you will be discovered.

That is the reason then why acts of kindness offer us the opportunity to learn how to live in the present. Always keep in mind the purpose of the mindfulness exercises is to learn ways of reducing stress in our lives. When stress is dissolved, we suddenly look at our bodies and are able to recognize symptoms don't seem to be present anymore. The causal connection between stress and symptoms is strong, but that does not mean it cannot be broken.

Dissolve that link with doing anonymous acts of kindness for the rest of the week.

May you secretive.
May you be sneaky.
May you have endless fun for the rest of the week.

Has your work on these exercises been stress free? Has it been helpful in reducing your symptoms? I certainly hope so! This is the primary reason I developed the mindfulness exercises in the first place.

If you struggled with pacing out these mindfulness exercises so as not to induce more stress, there are several Parkinsons Recovery programs that might help expedite your recovery. My Parkinsons Recovery Mindfulness Program sends the mindfulness exercises in an email to you each and every week. The initial exercise is sent to your email address on day one of the week and the deeper implications are sent four days later. The Parkinsons Recovery Mindfulness Program takes one full year to complete as each exercise is introduced one week at a time. For more information visit:

www.stress.parkinsonsrecovery.com

Parkinsons Recovery Memberships involve a variety of support websites that are essential to recovery. A difference mindfulness exercise is posted each week. For more information on Parkinsons Recovery memberships visit:

www.parkinsonsrecovery.org

Of course, the approach that works for many people is to purchase a single volume of the Parkinsons Recovery Mindfulness program at a time as you have already done! See the introduction for a listing of all nine Parkinsons Recovery Mindfulness volumes.

Thank you for Your Support

On behalf of the thousands of followers of Parkinsons Recovery, I want to thank you for your purchase of this booklet. One hundred percent (100%) of the profits purchases of my books and programs help subsidize the many free services I offer through Parkinsons Recovery -

www.parkinsonsrecovery.com

For information about other products, services and programs visit -

www.parkinsonsrecovery.me

www.ingramcontent.com/pod-product-compliance
Lightning Source LLC
Chambersburg PA
CBHW060226290526
45789CB00003B/1433